MINDFUL EATING AND WEIGHT MANAGEMENT

EHICHIOYA DOMINION

First Edition: February 2024

Library of Congress Cataloging-in-Publication Data:

Ehichioya Dominion

Mindful Eating and Weight Management

Designed by Ehichioya Dominion

Printed in Nigeria

Published by Ehichioya Dominion

No 33 off Osimen Street

Ekpoma, Edo State,

www.EhichioyadominionBooks.com

Cover design by Domi Gold

TABLE OF CONTENTS

B. Mindful Breathing Practices

C. Mindful Eating Journaling

D. Mindful Eating Exercises

VI. Incorporating Mindful Eating into Daily Life

A. Mindful Eating at Work

B. Mindful Eating for Social Gatherings

C. Mindful Snacking Habits

VII. Overcoming Challenges in Mindful Eating

A. Dealing with Emotional Eating

B. Handling Social Pressures

C. Addressing Common Mindful Eating Misconceptions

VIII. Mindful Movement and Exercise

A. Integrating Mindfulness into Physical Activity

B. The Role of Exercise in Overall Well-Being

IX. Mindful Eating Recipes and Meal Plans

A. Nutrient-Rich and Mindfully Prepared Recipes

B. Sample Mindful Eating Meal Plans

X. Tracking Progress and Setting Goals

A. Establishing Realistic Weight Management Goals

B. Using Mindfulness to Track Progress

C. Celebrating Achievements

<u>DESCRIPTION: MINDFUL EATING AND WEIGHT MANAGEMENT</u>

Embark on a transformative journey towards a healthier, more balanced lifestyle with our comprehensive guide, "Mindful Eating and Weight Management." This insightful ebook is a holistic exploration of mindful eating, weaving together the intricate connections between the mind and body to redefine your relationship with food.

INTRODUCTION: UNLOCKING THE POWER OF MINDFUL EATING FOR WEIGHT MANAGEMENT

Welcome to "Mindful Eating and Weight Management," a transformative journey towards achieving a harmonious balance between your mind, body, and the food you consume. In this groundbreaking eBook, we will explore the profound concept of mindful eating and its pivotal role in effective weight management.

DEFINITION OF MINDFUL EATING

Mindful eating goes beyond the act of consuming food; it is a conscious and intentional approach to nourishment that involves being fully present during every aspect of the eating experience. It invites you to engage with your meals in a way that fosters a deep connection with the flavors, textures, and sensations, ultimately leading to a heightened awareness of your body's signals.

OVERVIEW OF THE MIND-BODY CONNECTION

Our exploration begins with an understanding of the intricate relationship between the mind and body. Mindful eating is rooted in the recognition that our mental and emotional states significantly impact our eating habits. By cultivating mindfulness, we aim to foster a positive and intuitive connection between our thoughts, emotions, and the nourishment our bodies need.

IMPORTANCE OF MINDFUL EATING IN WEIGHT MANAGEMENT

Why is mindful eating essential for effective weight management? In this section, we delve into the significance of mindfulness in creating sustainable and healthy eating patterns. By embracing mindfulness, you embark on a holistic journey that transcends traditional diets, focusing on nourishment, satisfaction, and overall well-being.

As we progress through the subsequent chapters, you'll discover practical techniques, scientific insights, and actionable tips that will empower you to integrate mindful eating into your daily life. From understanding the difference between mindful and mindless eating to exploring the psychological and physiological impacts, each chapter is designed to equip you with the knowledge and tools needed for a transformative experience.

<u>CHAPTER II: UNDERSTANDING MINDFUL EATING</u>

In the pursuit of effective weight management, developing a profound understanding of mindful eating is paramount. This chapter will unravel the distinctions between mindful and mindless eating, dissect the key components of mindful eating, and shed light on the numerous benefits it bestows upon weight management.

A. MINDFUL VS. MINDLESS EATING

Mindful eating is a deliberate and conscious approach to consuming food, while mindless eating involves thoughtless and often automatic eating habits. Mindless eating can be influenced by external factors such as distractions, emotional triggers, and environmental cues. Recognizing the difference between the two is the first step towards fostering a healthier relationship with food.

B. COMPONENTS OF MINDFUL EATING

1. Awareness of Hunger and Fullness:

Mindful eating encourages tuning into your body's signals of hunger and fullness. By paying attention to the physical cues your body provides, you can distinguish between genuine hunger and emotional cravings. This awareness is pivotal in preventing overeating and promoting a balanced intake of nutrients.

2. Savoring Flavors and Textures:

Mindful eating invites you to engage your senses fully. Take the time to savor the flavors, textures, and aromas of your food. Appreciating the sensory aspects of eating not only enhances the dining experience but also helps in developing a greater satisfaction with smaller portions.

3. Eating with Intention and Attention:

Eating with intention means making conscious choices about what you consume, considering the nutritional value and how it aligns with your well-being goals. Eating with attention involves being fully present during meals, minimizing distractions, and focusing on the act of eating. This promotes a deeper connection with your food and facilitates better digestion.

C. BENEFITS OF MINDFUL EATING FOR WEIGHT MANAGEMENT

Mindful eating goes beyond the immediate act of consuming food; it offers a range of benefits that positively impact weight management:

Increased Awareness of Eating Habits: By paying attention to your eating patterns, you become more attuned to habits that may contribute to overeating or unhealthy choices.

Enhanced Portion Control: Mindful eating helps you recognize satiety cues, leading to better portion control and a reduced likelihood of overindulging.

Emotional Regulation: Mindful eating equips you with the tools to identify and address emotional triggers, reducing the tendency to turn to food for comfort.

Sustainable Weight Loss: Unlike restrictive diets, mindful eating fosters a sustainable approach to weight management, focusing on long-term habits rather than short-term fixes.

CHAPTER III: THE SCIENCE BEHIND MINDFUL EATING

Welcome to the scientific foundation of "Mindful Eating and Weight Management." In this chapter, we delve into the intricate mechanisms that underscore how mindful eating impacts digestion, metabolism, hormonal regulation, and the profound psychological effects it has on our food choices.

A. IMPACT ON DIGESTION AND METABOLISM

Understanding the Digestive Process:

Mindful eating serves as a catalyst for a well-coordinated digestive symphony. By engaging in mindful practices, such as savoring each bite and chewing thoroughly, you initiate a cascade of events that optimize the breakdown of nutrients. This enhanced digestion ensures that the body efficiently absorbs essential vitamins, minerals, and energy, contributing to overall metabolic health.

Elevating Metabolic Efficiency:

The mindful approach to eating extends its influence to metabolism. By being fully present during meals, you signal to your body that nourishment is a deliberate and conscious act. This heightened awareness activates metabolic processes, fostering efficiency in energy utilization. The result is a metabolism that operates optimally, aiding in weight management and promoting overall well-being.

B. HORMONAL REGULATION AND MINDFUL EATING

Balancing Ghrelin and Leptin Levels:

Mindful eating plays a pivotal role in modulating hunger and satiety hormones, such as ghrelin and leptin. By paying attention to your body's signals and eating with intention, you foster a more balanced hormonal environment. This balance reduces the likelihood of overeating, promoting healthier appetite regulation and contributing to weight management goals.

Stress Reduction and Cortisol Management:

Stress is a common factor in weight management challenges, often leading to increased cortisol levels. Mindful eating, coupled with stress reduction techniques, helps manage cortisol release. By addressing the psychological aspects of eating, you create a positive impact on hormonal regulation, promoting an environment conducive to weight management.

C. PSYCHOLOGICAL EFFECTS ON FOOD CHOICES

Breaking the Cycle of Emotional Eating:

Mindful eating serves as a powerful antidote to emotional eating. By cultivating awareness around emotional triggers, you can interrupt the automatic response of turning to food for comfort. Mindfulness empowers you to make conscious choices about how to respond to emotions, fostering healthier coping mechanisms beyond reaching for food.

Building a Positive Relationship with Food:

Psychologically, mindful eating facilitates the development of a positive relationship with food. It encourages a non-restrictive mindset, freeing you from the constraints of dieting. By approaching food with mindfulness, you can make choices aligned with your well-being, promoting a sustainable and joyful relationship with eating.

As we continue this exploration of mindful eating, practical strategies and exercises will be unveiled to help you integrate these scientific principles into your daily life. Join us on this enlightening journey to discover how the science of mindful eating can revolutionize your approach to weight management, creating a harmonious connection between your body, mind, and the food you consume.

CHAPTER IV: PRACTICAL TIPS FOR MINDFUL EATING

Embark on a journey to integrate mindful eating into your daily life with this chapter, which provides practical tips to enhance your awareness, create a mindful eating environment, engage your senses, and navigate emotional triggers.

A. MINDFUL MEAL PREPARATION

1. Conscious Ingredient Selection: Begin your mindful eating journey at the grocery store. Choose fresh, whole foods and be conscious of the nutritional value they bring to your meals.

2. Preparation as Meditation: Treat the act of preparing your meals as a mindful practice. Engage in the process, savoring the colors, textures, and scents of the ingredients.

3. Cooking with Intention: Infuse your cooking with positive intentions. Consider the nourishment you are providing to your body and the joy of creating a wholesome meal.

B. CREATING A PEACEFUL EATING ENVIRONMENT

1. Eliminate Distractions: Create a designated eating space free from distractions such as phones or electronic devices. This fosters a mindful environment focused on the act of eating.

2. Mindful Table Setting: Set a visually appealing table. Take a moment to appreciate the aesthetics, enhancing the overall dining experience.

3. Intentional Lighting and Ambiance: Adjust lighting and create a calming ambiance to promote a tranquil environment conducive to mindful eating.

C. USING ALL FIVE SENSES DURING MEALS

1. Sight: Admire the presentation of your meal. Notice the colors, shapes, and arrangement of the food on your plate.

2. Smell: Take a moment to inhale the aromas. Appreciate the scents of your meal before taking the first bite.

3. Touch: Engage your sense of touch by feeling the textures of your food. Notice the varying sensations as you chew.

4. Taste: Savor each flavor. Pay attention to the intricacies of taste, and linger on the experience.

5. Hearing: Be mindful of the sounds around you. Create a quiet atmosphere to allow for a more focused eating experience.

D. RECOGNIZING EMOTIONAL TRIGGERS AND RESPONSES

1. Mindful Emotional Check-ins: Before reaching for food, assess your emotional state. Are you truly hungry, or is there an emotional trigger prompting you to eat?

2. Alternative Coping Mechanisms: Identify non-food-related ways to address emotional needs. Practice deep breathing, take a short walk, or engage in a calming activity.

3. Mindful Eating Journal: Keep a journal to record your emotions and eating patterns. This self-reflection can unveil patterns and provide insights into emotional eating triggers.

By incorporating these practical tips into your daily routine, you pave the way for a more mindful approach to eating. These practices not only enhance the enjoyment of your meals but also contribute to a healthier relationship with food, aligning with your weight management goals. As we proceed, we will delve into specific mindful eating techniques to deepen your understanding and implementation of these practices.

CHAPTER V: MINDFUL EATING TECHNIQUES

Embark on a transformative journey with practical techniques that deepen your mindful eating experience. These exercises will guide you towards a heightened awareness of your body, breath, thoughts, and the sensory pleasures of eating.

A. BODY SCAN MEDITATION

Guided Awareness: Set aside a few moments for a body scan meditation. Start from the toes, gradually moving upward, paying attention to each part of your body. Notice sensations, tensions, or areas of relaxation. This practice enhances your awareness of the physical cues your body provides.

Integrating Mindfulness: As you scan each body part, breathe deeply and mindfully. Allow your breath to bring a sense of relaxation and presence to each area. The body scan meditation promotes a deeper connection between your mind and body, fostering a holistic approach to mindful eating.

B. MINDFUL BREATHING PRACTICES

Conscious Inhalation and Exhalation: Practice mindful breathing before meals. Inhale deeply, focusing on the breath filling your lungs, and exhale slowly, releasing tension. This conscious breathing brings you into the present moment, preparing your mind for a mindful eating experience.

Breath Awareness During Meals: While eating, periodically pause to take a few intentional breaths. Connect with your breath to maintain mindfulness throughout the meal. This practice helps prevent mindless eating and promotes a more deliberate and enjoyable dining experience.

C. MINDFUL EATING JOURNALING

Reflective Journaling: Keep a mindful eating journal to document your thoughts and feelings related to food. Record the foods you choose, your emotional state, and any physical sensations during meals. Reflect on patterns and connections between your mood and eating habits.

Gratitude Practice: Include a gratitude section in your journal. Express gratitude for the nourishment your food provides and the opportunity to engage in mindful eating. Cultivating gratitude enhances the positive emotional aspect of your relationship with food.

D. MINDFUL EATING EXERCISES

Sensory Exploration: Choose a small piece of food, such as a grape or piece of chocolate. Engage in a sensory exploration exercise, using all your senses to experience the food. Observe its color, feel its texture, smell its aroma, and savor its taste slowly. This exercise heightens your awareness and appreciation for each bite.

Mindful Chew and Pause: Practice mindful chewing by consciously chewing each bite thoroughly before swallowing. Pause between bites to assess your level of fullness and savor the flavors. This exercise helps prevent overeating and promotes a mindful, pleasurable eating experience.

As we delve into these mindful eating techniques, you'll discover how integrating these practices into your daily routine enhances your overall well-being and contributes to effective weight management. These techniques lay the foundation for a mindful approach to eating that extends beyond individual meals, creating a sustainable and fulfilling lifestyle.

CHAPTER VI: INCORPORATING MINDFUL EATING INTO DAILY LIFE

Mindful eating is not just a practice; it's a way of life. Explore how to seamlessly integrate mindfulness into your daily routine, whether you're at work, attending social gatherings, or navigating snacking habits.

A. MINDFUL EATING AT WORK

1. Lunchtime Rituals: Designate time for a mindful lunch break. Step away from your work environment, savor your meal without distractions, and use this time as a mental reset.

2. Conscious Snacking: Opt for nourishing snacks and be intentional about your snacking habits. Choose nutrient-dense options and practice mindful consumption, avoiding mindless munching at your desk.

3. Mindful Meetings: During work meetings that involve food, be present with your eating. Slow down, engage your senses, and appreciate the flavors. This not only promotes mindfulness but also enhances your overall work experience.

B. MINDFUL EATING FOR SOCIAL GATHERINGS

1. Pre-Event Awareness: Before attending social gatherings, take a moment to check in with your hunger levels. This awareness allows you to approach the event with a balanced mindset, making mindful choices.

2. Strategic Plate Selection: Survey the available food options before loading your plate. Choose a variety of items mindfully, focusing on balance and moderation.

3. Conscious Conversation: Engage in conversations that go beyond food. Enjoy the social aspect of the gathering, shifting the focus from eating to connecting with others.

C. MINDFUL SNACKING HABITS

1. Snack Planning: Plan your snacks mindfully, considering both taste and nutritional value. Have pre-portioned snacks readily available to avoid impulsive choices.

2. Savoring Small Bites: When snacking, savor each bite as you would during a meal. Pay attention to flavors and textures, and take your time to enjoy the experience.

3. Mindful Snack Breaks: Incorporate short breaks into your day for mindful snacking. Step away from your routine, focus on your snack, and allow it to serve as a moment of relaxation and rejuvenation.

As you navigate daily life, these mindful eating practices contribute to a sustainable and enjoyable approach to nutrition. By incorporating mindfulness into work, social events, and snacking, you cultivate a balanced relationship with food that aligns with your weight management goals. In the following chapters, we'll address challenges that may arise and explore how to extend mindfulness beyond eating to create a holistic and balanced lifestyle.

CHAPTER VII: OVERCOMING CHALLENGES IN MINDFUL EATING

Embarking on a mindful eating journey may come with its own set of challenges. In this chapter, we address common obstacles and provide strategies to overcome them, ensuring a successful integration of mindfulness into your eating habits.

A. DEALING WITH EMOTIONAL EATING

1. Cultivating Emotional Awareness: Recognize and acknowledge your emotions without judgment. Practice mindfulness to become aware of emotional triggers that may lead to eating. Pause and assess whether your hunger is physical or emotionally driven.

2. Developing Alternative Coping Strategies: Establish a repertoire of non-food-related coping mechanisms for dealing with stress, sadness, or boredom. Engage in activities such as meditation, deep breathing, or a short walk to redirect your focus and manage emotions without resorting to emotional eating.

3. Mindful Eating in Emotional Moments: If emotional eating does occur, approach it with compassion rather than self-criticism. Practice mindfulness even during emotional moments, being present with your food choices and savoring each bite.

B. HANDLING SOCIAL PRESSURES

1. Communicating Mindful Choices: Communicate your mindful eating goals to friends and family. Educate them about your journey and the importance of being mindful about food choices. This can help alleviate social pressures to overindulge.

2. Navigating Social Events: Plan ahead for social gatherings by setting intentions and deciding in advance how you'll approach the event. Focus on enjoying the social aspect rather than solely the food.

3. Respecting Personal Boundaries: Politely but firmly communicate your boundaries when faced with well-meaning but insistent offers of food. Remember that it's okay to decline or have smaller portions in social settings.

C. ADDRESSING COMMON MINDFUL EATING MISCONCEPTIONS

1. Understanding the Learning Curve: Mindful eating is a skill that takes time to develop. Be patient with yourself as you navigate through the learning curve, understanding that consistency is key to its effectiveness.

2. Dispelling All-or-Nothing Thinking: Mindful eating doesn't require perfection. Avoid the trap of all-or-nothing thinking and embrace the gradual integration of mindful practices into your eating routine.

3. Customizing Mindful Practices: Mindful eating is a personal journey. Tailor the techniques to suit your preferences and lifestyle. Experiment with different practices to find what works best for you.

As you encounter these challenges, remember that overcoming them is a part of the mindful eating process. By developing resilience and applying the strategies provided, you'll navigate these hurdles with grace, fostering a positive relationship with food that aligns with your weight management goals. In the following chapters, we'll explore the role of mindful movement and exercise, delve into mindful recipes, and discuss how to maintain a balanced and mindful lifestyle beyond eating.

CHAPTER VIII: MINDFUL MOVEMENT AND EXERCISE

Explore the symbiotic relationship between mindfulness and physical activity, understanding how integrating mindfulness into your exercise routine contributes to overall well-being.

A. INTEGRATING MINDFULNESS INTO PHYSICAL ACTIVITY

1. Conscious Warm-Up: Begin your exercise routine with a mindful warm-up. Pay attention to the movements of your body, the sensations, and your breath. This primes your mind for a focused and intentional workout.

2. Mindful Cardiovascular Exercise: Whether running, walking, or cycling, infuse mindfulness into your cardiovascular workout. Be present with each step, focusing on your breath, the rhythm of your movements, and the environment around you.

3. Weight Training with Intention: Approach weight training with a mindful mindset. Engage in each repetition with purpose, concentrating on the muscle groups you're working. Connect your mind to the physical exertion, fostering a deeper mind-body connection.

B. THE ROLE OF EXERCISE IN OVERALL WELL-BEING

1. Holistic Health Benefits: Understand that exercise extends beyond physical health, influencing mental and emotional well-being. Regular physical activity has been linked to reduced stress, improved mood, and enhanced cognitive function.

2. Enhanced Mind-Body Connection: Exercise serves as a powerful tool for reinforcing the mind-body connection. Mindful movement not only contributes to physical fitness but also cultivates mental clarity and emotional resilience.

3. Stress Reduction through Movement: Engage in activities like yoga or tai chi that combine mindful movement with meditative elements. These practices not only improve flexibility and strength but also serve as effective stress-reducing exercises.

As you infuse mindfulness into your physical activity, you'll discover that exercise becomes a holistic practice contributing to your overall well-being. In the upcoming chapters, we will explore mindful eating recipes, meal plans, and discuss how to set realistic goals while tracking progress. This holistic approach ensures that mindfulness permeates every aspect of your life, promoting a balanced and sustainable lifestyle that aligns with your weight management objectives.

<u>CHAPTER IX: MINDFUL EATING RECIPES AND MEAL PLANS</u>

Delve into a collection of nutrient-rich and mindfully prepared recipes, as well as sample meal plans designed to nourish both your body and your mindfulness practice.

A. NUTRIENT-RICH AND MINDFULLY PREPARED RECIPES

1. Mango Avocado Quinoa Bowl: Explore the vibrant flavors of a quinoa bowl with ripe mango, creamy avocado, cherry tomatoes, and a drizzle of citrus dressing. This recipe combines nutrient-rich ingredients to satisfy both taste buds and nutritional needs.

2. Baked Salmon with Lemon and Dill: Elevate your protein intake with a delicious baked salmon dish. Infused with the freshness of lemon and dill, this recipe not only provides omega-3 fatty acids but also invites a mindful cooking experience.

3. Vegetarian Stir-Fry with Ginger Sesame Sauce: Immerse yourself in the colors and textures of a vegetable stir-fry featuring broccoli, bell peppers, snap peas, and tofu. The ginger sesame sauce adds a flavorful touch, turning a simple stir-fry into a mindful culinary experience.

B. SAMPLE MINDFUL EATING MEAL PLANS

DAY 1: MINDFUL BEGINNING

- **Breakfast:** Overnight oats with mixed berries and a sprinkle of chia seeds.

- **Lunch:** Grilled chicken salad with a variety of colorful vegetables and a light vinaigrette.

- **Dinner:** Quinoa-stuffed bell peppers with black beans, corn, and a side of roasted sweet potatoes.

DAY 2: BALANCING ACT

- **Breakfast:** Greek yogurt parfait with granola, sliced bananas, and a drizzle of honey.

- **Lunch:** Brown rice bowl with sautéed spinach, chickpeas, cherry tomatoes, and a tahini dressing.

- **Dinner:** Baked cod with a lemon herb crust, accompanied by steamed asparagus and quinoa.

DAY 3: MINDFUL INDULGENCE

- **Breakfast:** Whole grain pancakes topped with mixed berries and a dollop of Greek yogurt.

- **Lunch:** Lentil and vegetable soup with a side of whole-grain bread.

- **Dinner:** Zucchini noodles with tomato and basil sauce, served alongside a colorful side salad.

These meal plans incorporate a variety of nutrient-dense foods while embracing the principles of mindful eating. The recipes are designed to not only nourish your body but also engage your senses, fostering a deeper connection with the act of eating. In the following chapters, we'll explore how to set and track realistic weight management goals and extend mindfulness beyond eating to create a balanced and mindful lifestyle.

CHAPTER X: TRACKING PROGRESS AND SETTING GOALS

Explore the art of setting realistic weight management goals, employing mindfulness as a tool to track your progress, and celebrating the achievements along your mindful eating journey.

A. ESTABLISHING REALISTIC WEIGHT MANAGEMENT GOALS

1. Mindful Goal Setting: Introduce the concept of setting mindful, realistic, and achievable goals. Encourage readers to move beyond numbers on a scale and focus on holistic well-being, including physical health, mental clarity, and emotional balance.

2. Smart Goals: Break down the process of goal-setting using the SMART criteria - Specific, Measurable, Achievable, Relevant, and Time-bound. This approach helps individuals create clear and attainable objectives.

3. Non-Scale Victories: Emphasize the significance of recognizing non-scale victories, such as improved energy levels, better sleep quality, or enhanced mood. These victories contribute to an overall sense of well-being beyond mere weight metrics.

B. USING MINDFULNESS TO TRACK PROGRESS

1. Mindful Journaling: Introduce the practice of mindful journaling to track eating patterns, emotional triggers, and moments of mindfulness. Encourage readers to reflect on their experiences, fostering self-awareness and understanding.

2. Mindful Eating Logs: Provide templates for mindful eating logs, where individuals can record their meals, emotions, and sensations associated with eating. This tool helps in identifying patterns and making mindful adjustments.

3. Body Awareness Practices: Guide readers through body awareness exercises, helping them tune in to physical sensations, hunger cues, and the mind-body connection. Mindful awareness contributes to making informed choices aligned with health goals.

C. CELEBRATING ACHIEVEMENTS

1. Mindful Reflection: Encourage regular reflection on progress, acknowledging both small and significant achievements. Mindfulness enables individuals to appreciate the journey, fostering a positive relationship with their bodies and efforts.

2. Mindful Celebrations: Suggest celebrating milestones with non-food-related rewards, such as a self-care day, a nature walk, or a mindful meditation session. Mindful celebrations reinforce the connection between achievements and well-being.

3. Community Support: Highlight the importance of seeking support from a community or a mindful eating group. Sharing successes creates a positive atmosphere and reinforces the idea that the mindful eating journey is a collective and encouraging experience.

By approaching weight management goals with mindfulness, individuals not only enhance their chances of success but also cultivate a deeper understanding of their bodies and minds. The next chapter will explore extending mindfulness beyond eating, applying it to various aspects of life to create a balanced and mindful lifestyle.

CHAPTER XI: MINDFUL LIVING BEYOND EATING

Explore the extension of mindfulness principles beyond eating, integrating them into various aspects of life to create a balanced and mindful lifestyle.

A. APPLYING MINDFULNESS TO OTHER ASPECTS OF LIFE

1. Mindful Daily Rituals: Encourage incorporating mindfulness into daily routines such as waking up, commuting, or winding down. Discuss how simple practices like mindful breathing or brief moments of reflection can enhance overall well-being.

2. Mindful Communication: Explore the role of mindfulness in effective communication. Highlight the importance of being present and attentive in conversations, fostering deeper connections with others.

3. Mindful Work Habits: Discuss the application of mindfulness in the workplace, promoting focus, stress reduction, and enhanced productivity. Share techniques for incorporating short mindfulness practices during the workday.

B. CREATING A BALANCED AND MINDFUL LIFESTYLE

1. Holistic Well-Being: Emphasize the interconnectedness of physical, mental, and emotional well-being. Encourage readers to cultivate a mindful approach to health that considers nutrition, exercise, sleep, and stress management.

2. Mindful Leisure Activities: Explore the role of mindfulness in leisure pursuits. Discuss how engaging in activities like nature walks, art, or hobbies with a mindful attitude can contribute to a more balanced and enjoyable life.

3. Digital Mindfulness: Address the impact of technology on well-being and provide tips for mindful technology use. Discuss the importance of unplugging, setting boundaries, and being present in the digital age.

By extending mindfulness principles beyond eating, individuals can create a more harmonious and fulfilling lifestyle. The final chapter will recap key concepts, provide encouragement for continued mindful practices, and offer final thoughts on long-term weight management.

CHAPTER XII: CONCLUSION

A. RECAP OF KEY CONCEPTS

Throughout this journey of exploring mindful eating and weight management, we've delved into the core principles that define this approach. From distinguishing mindful vs. mindless eating to understanding the components of mindful eating—awareness of hunger and fullness, savoring flavors, and eating with intention—we've built a foundation for cultivating a more conscious relationship with food.

In the exploration of the science behind mindful eating, we've uncovered its impact on digestion, metabolism, hormonal regulation, and the profound psychological effects on food choices. Practical tips, mindful eating techniques, and the integration of mindfulness into daily life have provided actionable steps for readers seeking a holistic approach to well-being.

B. ENCOURAGEMENT FOR CONTINUED MINDFUL EATING PRACTICE

As you embark on or continue your mindful eating journey, remember that transformation is a gradual process. Embrace the small victories, be patient with setbacks, and recognize the power of consistency. Cultivate mindfulness not just during meals but in all aspects of your life. Let it become a guiding force for creating a healthier, more balanced lifestyle.

Mindful eating is not a destination but a lifelong practice. Each moment offers an opportunity to bring awareness and intention into your choices, fostering a deeper connection with yourself and your surroundings. Celebrate the ongoing commitment to mindfulness and the positive impact it has on your overall well-being.

C. FINAL THOUGHTS ON LONG-TERM WEIGHT MANAGEMENT

Long-term weight management isn't solely about numbers on a scale; it's about nourishing your body, mind, and soul. Mindful eating provides a sustainable approach, addressing not just what you eat but how and why you eat. By incorporating mindfulness into your daily life, you're not only fostering a healthy relationship with food but also laying the groundwork for a balanced and fulfilling existence.

Remember, the journey to long-term well-being is unique for each individual. Embrace your personal path, stay attuned to your body's signals, and savor the richness that mindful living can bring to every aspect of your life. May your continued mindful practices guide you on a journey of lasting health, happiness, and self-discovery.